Aging - Slow Down Getting Old With These 8 Actionable Tips

Stay Younger Looking By Minimizing the Effects of Growing Old

Ron Kness

https://SecretsofAging.net

Contents

Disclaimer

We hope you enjoy reading our report however we do suggest you read our disclaimer. All the material written in this report is provided for informational purposes only and is general in nature.

Every person is a unique individual and what has worked for some or even many may not work for you. Any information perceived as advice by must be considered in light of your own particular set of circumstances.

The author or person sharing this information does not assume any responsibility for the accuracy or outcome of your use of the content.

Every attempt has been made to provide well researched and up to date content at the time of writing. Now all the legalities have been taken care of, please enjoy the content.

Introduction

As you read this publication you will recognize a great truth – that while aging is inevitable, its effects are not. There are ways the effects from aging can be either slowed down or in some cases reversed. A quick look at people around you will show that apparent age and chronological age are not the same thing.

Some people look much younger than their years, others much older. Why the difference?

Some genetically-predisposed factors that may delay our apparent aging or otherwise are beyond our control. There is an increasing wave of information that shows conclusively that we as individuals have much more control over our rate of aging than we have been previously told.

For those who are prepared to accept this and take personal action to support it, this is incredibly empowering. Each of us has the ability, through daily mindful choices, to delay our apparent rate of aging relative to our actual age.

We can add years to our life. In all those extra years and those that precede them, we can add joy and vitality to our daily life. We can delay the effects of aging on our physical, mental and emotional selves, and look younger doing it.

Fighting the good fight against the effects of aging is much more about prevention than cure. The choices are ours. Let's get started ….

Your Skin as You Age

There are several factors that affect the quality of our skin as we grow older. Some of these factors are beyond our control, such as our chronological or actual age and genetics, but it's also great to know that some aspects are within our power to change or influence.

Lifestyle and diet are the major significant influencing factors, but before you make any changes for the sake of your skin health and appearance, it pays to understand the aging process of your skin.

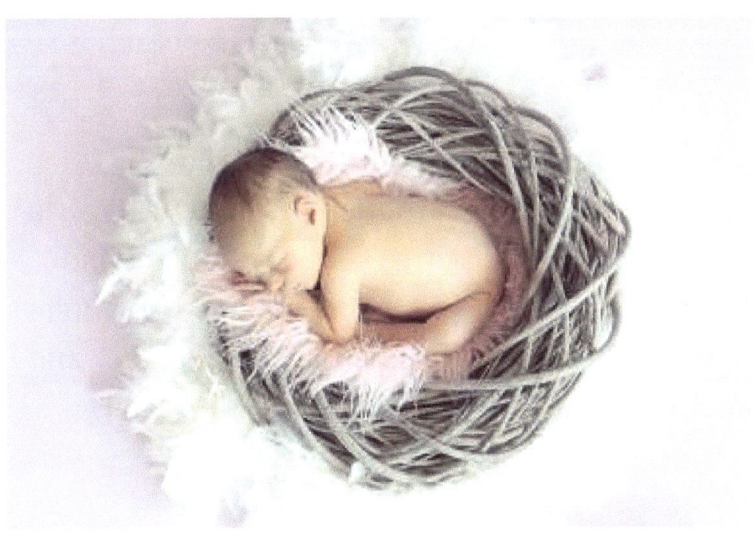

In Your 40's

Once you are in the 40's age group, the lymphatic system tends to slow down, just like most of the organs and systems inside your body. Unfortunately, this system also plays a vital role in getting rid of toxins from the body.

This decline in the ability to remove toxins as efficiently as before can result in the breaking down of the elastic fibers that are important for supporting the lymph glands. What you will notice as a result is a puffy look around your cheeks and eyes.

It is also during your 40's that your sebum production may decline and this can adversely impact the outer protective coating of the skin making it more sensitive to environmental influences.

These changes are also accompanied by fluctuating estrogen production, which can cause visible signs of the skin looking less radiant and firm. It can also lead to the appearance of wrinkles and the start of sagging skin around the neck and décolletage area.

If your eyes begin to look a little sunken, this can also be due to bone loss caused by the reduced estrogen production.

In Your 50's

Now your life is just beginning! So too is a significant drop in collagen production! This is why your skin begins to seriously sag. At this stage of life you may notice the appearance of little pigmentation changes on the skin's surface. Age spots may start to appear on your face, arms and especially the back of your hands.

These skin blemishes can also be accompanied by the presence of spider veins which are caused by damaged blood vessels. It is also in your 50's that your skin pores can increase in size. This is because your skin loosens making the openings of the pores appear bigger.

Some women, especially fair-skinned women, may experience drier, flakier skin with more wrinkles, than other women who have naturally oilier or darker pigmentation.

Facial hair may also begin to be a problem, because of the hormonal imbalances taking place.

The decline of estrogen production and the decline of collagen leads to a lack of skin moisture and 'luster' loss. Therefore, your skin's elasticity isn't so springy anymore either!

It is also during this period of a woman's life that the skin becomes more prone to inflammation.

In Your 60's

In the next decade some of your hormones may now start to return to their normal levels. So there is good news after all!

However, your fascia, the part that connects your bone to your skin may begin to deteriorate, thereby contributing to an increasing loss of your natural skin tone.

So what is the good news if this happens? The good news is your skin sensitivity may lessen, compared to previous years. If your skin displayed patchy red areas, it too may begin to appear less discolored.

At this stage, your blood circulation to the skin may tend to decline and this can significantly make your skin look duller. Your lips may become thinner and any wrinkles around the mouth may become more apparent.

To sum it all up – changes to your skin are inevitable as you age, however, the rate of change can be minimized by your actions. Your major concerns regarding skin health as you age should be a focus on a healthy diet and avoidance of dietary and environmental toxins.

Drink plenty of fresh water to keep your skin well-hydrated at all times, stick to your skin firming rituals and get your necessary sun exposure early in the day.

A Healthy Lifestyle Equals a Longer Life

Healthy lifestyle habits certainly help us live longer, that's only natural. If we don't abuse our bodies, we won't wear them out as quickly as they might otherwise.

This is proven scientifically, as experts have found that if you improve your health at a cellular level, you are also improving your cellular age and reducing the rate of decline.

However, it also makes sense that the opposite is true. If you lead an unhealthy lifestyle and abuse your health, damage which occurs cell by cell adds up to an increased rate of apparent aging. You are essentially speeding up the aging process, harming your health and reducing your longevity.

Men's Lifestyle Habits and Prostate Cancer

A research study revealed a link between men's lifestyle habits and their risk of prostate cancer. The study involved 35 male participants over a five-year period and focused on the early diagnosis of prostate cancer.

This study showed that following a healthy diet and exercising regularly helped improve the length of 'telomeres'. Telomeres are the protective caps found at the end of each chromosome that play a crucial role in regulating the lifespan of cells.

The shortening of telomeres causes certain cells to die earlier than they would otherwise, if a healthier lifestyle was followed.

Some of the male study participants made positive changes to their lifestyle by eating a healthy diet, exercising on a regular basis and indulging in stress-reduction activities such as meditation and yoga. They also joined a support group.

The results showed that these men were found to have a 10% increase in their telomeres length. In the control group were 25 men who did not make any changes to their lifestyle habits. Their telomeres decreased in length by up to 3% and they also were diagnosed with early stage prostate cancer. The results of this study were published in the Lancet Oncology.

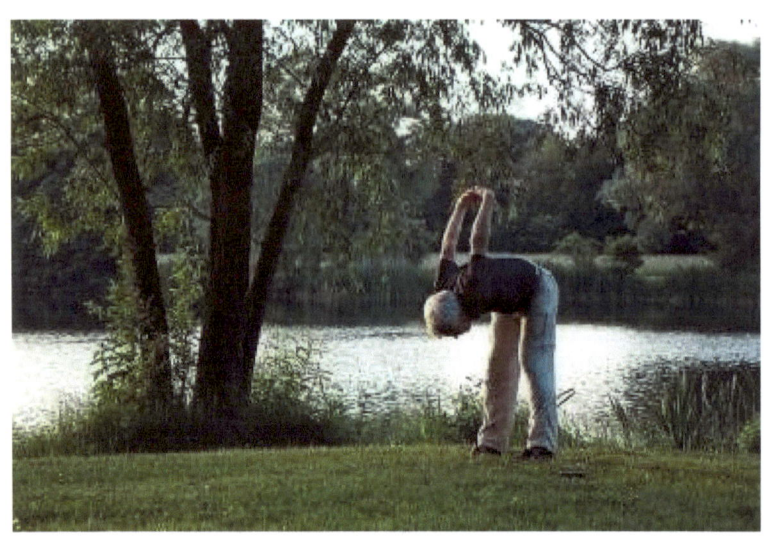

An Unhealthy Lifestyle Equals A Shorter Life

Although the number of incidences of people suffering from chronic illnesses such as obesity, cancer, stroke, arthritis and heart disease is increasing, experts agree that these conditions can almost always be controlled or prevented through healthy lifestyle habits.

In line with this claim, researchers from the University of Zurich conducted a study on the effects of 4 factors and how it affected their life expectancy. These four factors were:

1. Being sedentary
2. Following an unhealthy diet
3. Cigarette smoking

4. Excessive alcohol consumption

While each of these factors contributes to a decrease in life expectancy, combining them greatly compounds the effect. The results of this study showed that a person whose lifestyle included all 4 risk factors had at least twice the mortality risk of those who did not involve any.

This finding was based on data gathered from a study of 16,721 people from 1977 to 2008. As the data sample and the time-frame were large, researchers consider the results very conclusive.

The researchers found that 75-year-old individuals who didn't partake in the four negative lifestyle choices had up to a 67% probability of surviving for the next ten years.

Those statistics are definitely worth thinking about if you don't follow a healthy lifestyle. Taking action to remove negative factors from your lifestyle can result in a longer lifespan and an improved quality of life to enjoy it with.

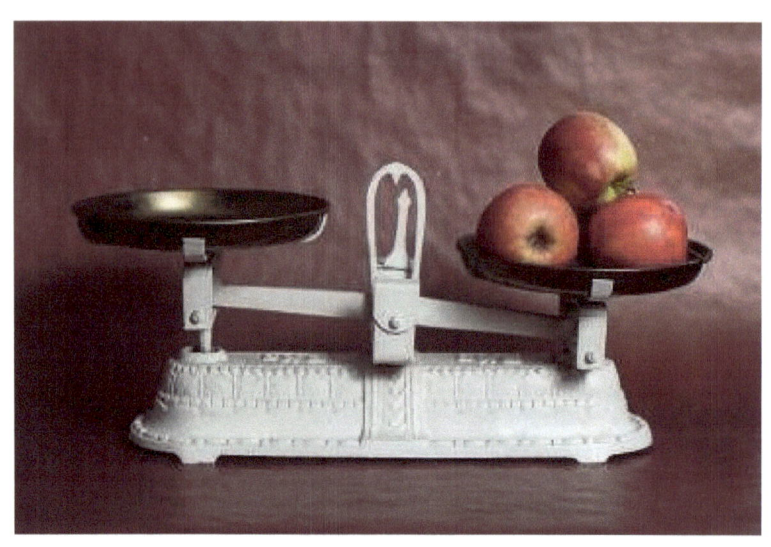

Aging and the 'Middle-Age Spread'

The phrase 'middle-age spread', by its own definition, is considered synonymous with aging. Unfortunately, for too many it has become an accepted part of life and growing older. It is as if we believe it is normal or inevitable, rather than a dangerous sign of poor lifestyle choices.

Distinguishing Subcutaneous Fat from Visceral Fat

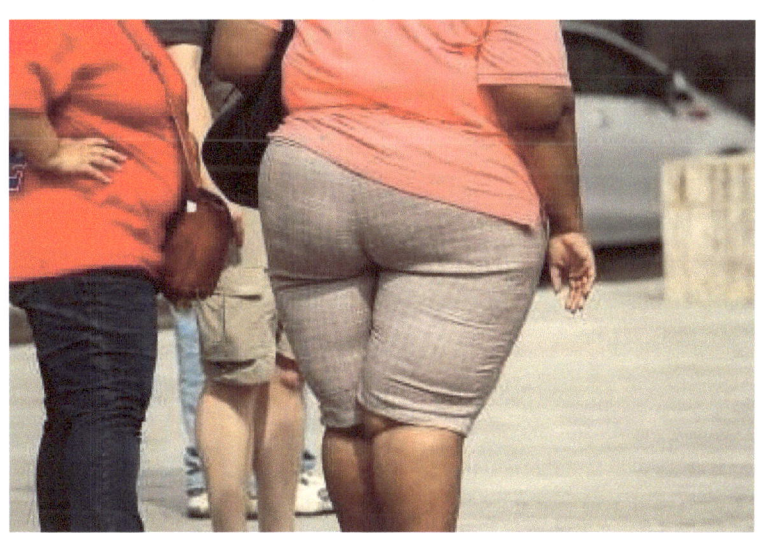

Abdominal fat is also referred to as 'visceral' fat. If you have excess abdominal fat, you should do something about it

... and the sooner the better. Abdominal fat has been linked to many health risks. Health professionals and organizations use waistline measurements as one indicator when performing health checkups.

Although subcutaneous fat is not as dangerous as visceral fat, neither of these should ever be allowed to accumulate in the midriff area.

Subcutaneous fat is the kind you can grasp or pinch with your hands, located just below the skin. Visceral fat is much more dangerous to your health than subcutaneous fat.

Visceral fat is located deep within the body's abdominal cavity, out of hands reach. Excessive amounts of visceral fat have been linked to different kinds of metabolic disorders, type 2 diabetes, breast cancer, gallbladder problems and cardiovascular disease.

While where the fat accumulates in the body is partly determined by hormones, gender and genes, it also reflects a person's lifestyle habits and choices.

The Dangers of Abdominal Fat

Studies reveal that abdominal fat cells are biologically active and any excess can significantly disrupt the normal functioning and balance of hormones.

Abdominal fat releases cytokines which are immune system chemicals, which can increase the risk of cardiovascular diseases. The release of these bio-chemicals can also affect the body's insulin sensitivity and it may lead to blood pressure issues and blood clotting.

Another reason why visceral fat can be dangerous to your health is due to its proximity to the portal vein. The portal vein is responsible for carrying blood from the intestinal area into the liver.

When visceral fat releases substances such as free fatty acids, they are carried into the portal vein and then travel to the liver, affecting the production of blood lipids.

An increase in the amount of visceral fat equates to increased insulin resistance, higher levels of the bad LDL cholesterol and lower levels of the good HDL cholesterol.

Visceral fat has also been shown to secrete proteins that contribute to the development of atherosclerosis, which is a condition that leads to clogged arteries. This puts the person at a higher risk of having a heart attack.

How to Stop the Middle-Age Spread

If you are around middle age, living an unhealthy lifestyle, dining on processed foods, sitting in front of the television or computer all day, drinking high volumes of soft drink and/or alcohol, you will most likely be able to look down and see your very own 'middle-age spread'.

Avoiding any physical activity and eating a diet high in carbohydrates is a surefire way to a bigger belly and putting yourself at a higher risk of lifestyle diseases.

A study showed that exercising vigorously for eight consecutive months helped participants reduce their visceral fat by as much as 8%. This may sound great to some people, but just watching what you eat and reducing your sugary, high carb foods can reduce that bulge even quicker than exercise can!

Sit-ups and other spot exercises may help in tightening the abdominal muscles, but it can't reach visceral fat. Getting rid of excessive abdominal fat isn't possible without paying attention to your eating habits. Plain and simple. So steer clear of refined grains, pasta, fizzy beverages, high sodium and sugary foods.

Instead, fill your body with real whole foods, such as fruits, vegetables, fish and meat that hasn't been processed. You can start your day with an egg or two, instead of pancakes and syrup.

Making that one simple change will help reduce your midriff bulge, making you feel and look better too!

Keep A Pet for Mental and Physical Health

'Pets as therapy'. This is a phrase that you may have heard and with good reason. Pets are excellent for keeping us healthy and are often used as therapy, especially for those getting on in years.

Of course, you don't have to be older to benefit from having a pet around. It's just that as we age, or enter our maturing years, a pet helps to keep a greater focus on the now. Many elderly citizens worry about their future, their tomorrow. What if it doesn't come? A pet, by its needs and its actions, helps to keep them thinking of 'right now'.

Having this mindset is particularly helpful for those who are battling with a disease. Their thoughts of tomorrow may bring fear and unnecessary worry. These feelings of anxiousness can hugely decrease or even cease to exist once they start caring for a pet.

This is a major reason why owning a pet can help you stay mentally and emotionally healthy in your latter years.

Increased Chances for Physical Activity

If a person has a dog, chances are they are going to take it for a walk. Therefore, their physical activity will be stimulated to a much higher degree than if they keep a goldfish.

However, regardless of what type of pet a person has, they still must care for it. So they still have to get up and do something, although exertion levels will vary depending on the pet.

Better Ability to Cope with Anxiety

Elderly and psychiatric patients who are pet owners have been found to be more capable of managing their anxiety. This is part of the reason why several nursing homes have started to incorporate an animal program, or as stated before, using 'pets as therapy', which allows elderly residents to own a pet.

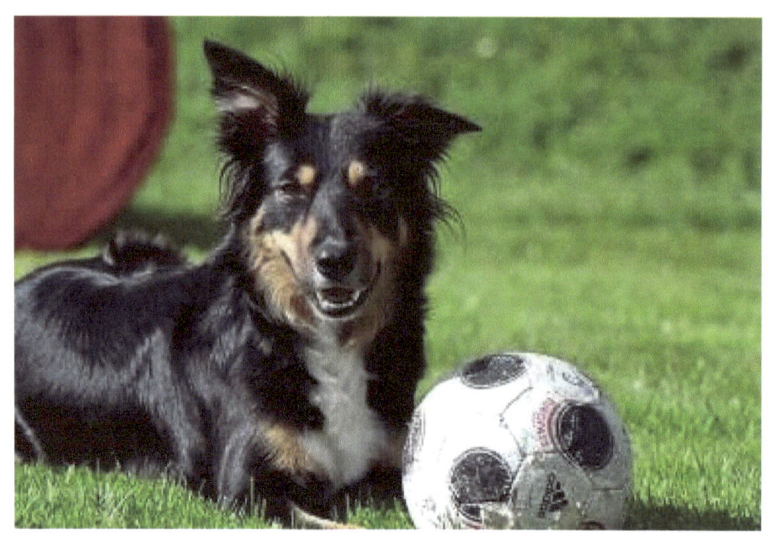

Improved Ability to Tolerate Social Isolation

Elderly citizens who own pets face lower risks of depression because their pets help them better tolerate social isolation. This is especially true for seniors who have a mobility problem and live on their own.

For elderly pet owners, having a pet means having a great companion who provides them with friendship and unconditional love that they may no longer receive from their fellow human beings.

This may be due to reduced opportunities for social contact. Reasons can include outliving peers and simply a lack of interest from friends or family.

Many researchers agree that the most serious ailment that an elderly person can have is not heart disease, diabetes or cancer, but loneliness.

When loneliness starts to engulf an elderly person's home, their depressed state makes them much more vulnerable to any medical condition.

Lowered Risk of Heart Disease

Being a pet owner leads to both a lowered risk of stress and an increased rate of survival from a heart attack.

Experts have found that pets help stroke victims recover more quickly as they find strength from their pet's presence. A survey was conducted where over 5,000 people underwent cardiovascular checkups and evaluations.

The pet owners showed significantly lower risks of symptoms linked to cardiovascular disease.

Owning and caring for a pet is an excellent way of helping to stay mentally, emotionally and physically healthy as you age, while giving and receiving love at the same time.

A Healthy Sex Life as You Age

It has been a common belief that sexual desire decreases as we age, however that does not have to be so! Research reveals that an individual's sexual desires, actions and thoughts, continue throughout their lifetime. Sex is not designed to be limited to the younger population.

A Healthy Sex Life Promotes Optimal Health

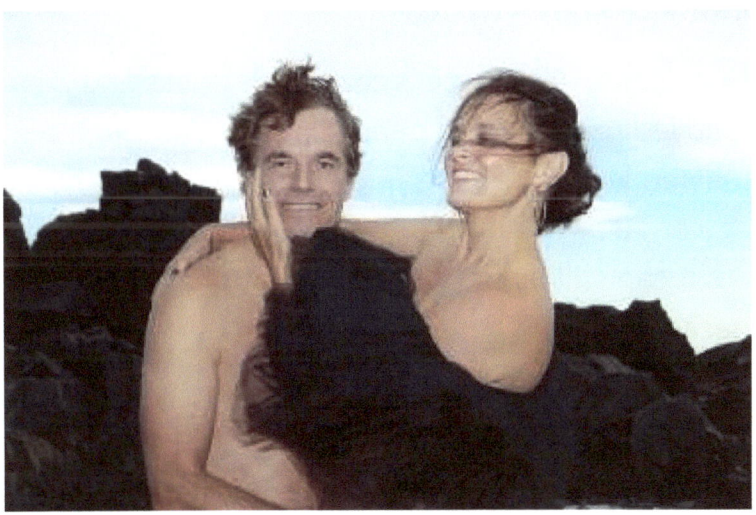

Human touch is an important aspect of one's sex life that evokes feelings of joy, affection, intimacy, passion and romance which makes it a powerful emotional experience.

A healthy sex life is important for maintaining, improving and preserving a person's physical, emotional and psychological health.

A survey commissioned by the National Council on Aging showed that almost half of the elderly or senior population surveyed acknowledged engaging in sexual activities at least once a month. They also claimed that their sex life had improved with age and that their sexual satisfaction was higher or equal to that of when they were in their 40's.

Intimacy Knows No Age

Our need for intimacy is certainly ageless and is enjoyed regardless of gender or age. Although sex may no longer be the same when you reach the age of 70 or 80 compared to when you were 20 or 30, it can still be better in your senior years. This is because you are wiser, experienced and more aware of you and your partner's needs.

As an older adult, you are now free from the unrealistic ideals that are often present in youth. You are no longer limited by the prejudices of other people. Also, your own children have grown and you now have more liberty to relax and enjoy each other's company, in your own time.

The Road Blocks to a Healthy Sex Life

Too many adults worry about their sex life as they age. These worries spring from the effects of aging to their physical appearance and the concern of their sexual performance.

These thoughts may cause them to avoid any sexual encounters altogether. This then affects not only their sex life but their emotional and psychological health as well. Unfortunately, of course, there are individuals whose sex life is negatively affected by their medical conditions or the loss of their loved one.

It doesn't matter what age you are, having or enjoying a healthy sex life is good for you! If there is something that is stopping you, it is time to look at the reason and see if you can address the problem.

The first step is honest appraisal of your situation. Are the limiting factors physical or emotional? If you are constrained by physical limitations, talk to your doctor. However, even physiological issues quite often have an underlying emotional basis.

Take time to understand yourself and your reasons. Be open and brave enough to discuss it with you partner and if appropriate, with a trusted counselor such as your family doctor.

Arm yourself with the right information and be proactive about your sexual health. Your 'mental health' and 'joy of life' is greatly affected by it. If you think you need professional help, then do not hesitate to do so.

An aging body should not deprive you of the opportunity to explore the exciting and sensual aspects of your own sexuality.

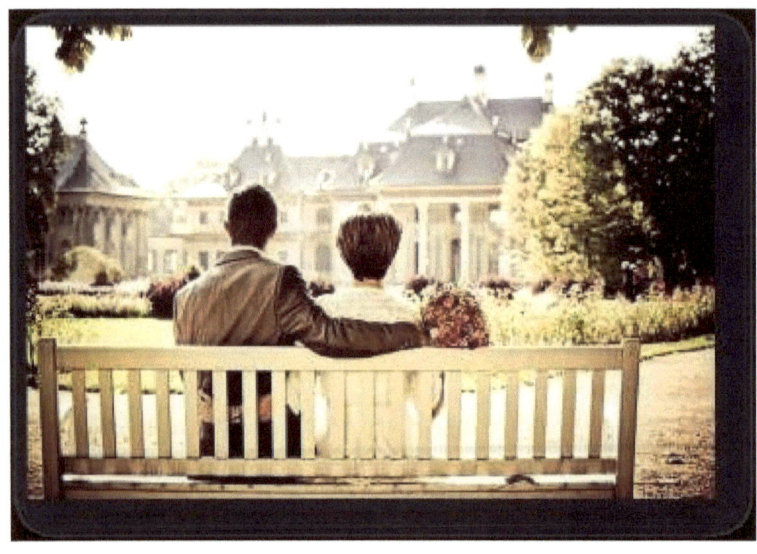

Does Diabetes Accelerate Aging?

We are being made increasingly aware that diabetes is a growing health problem. Although diabetes is increasingly more prevalent in the young, it is one of the most common age-related illnesses.

It is not too long ago that type 2 diabetes was almost unheard of in younger people. This correlation led to the assumption that type 2 diabetes was caused by the aging process. Increased understanding of the true cause of it, and the increasing incidence in young people, has turned that thinking around. It now begs the question – does diabetes accelerate the aging process?

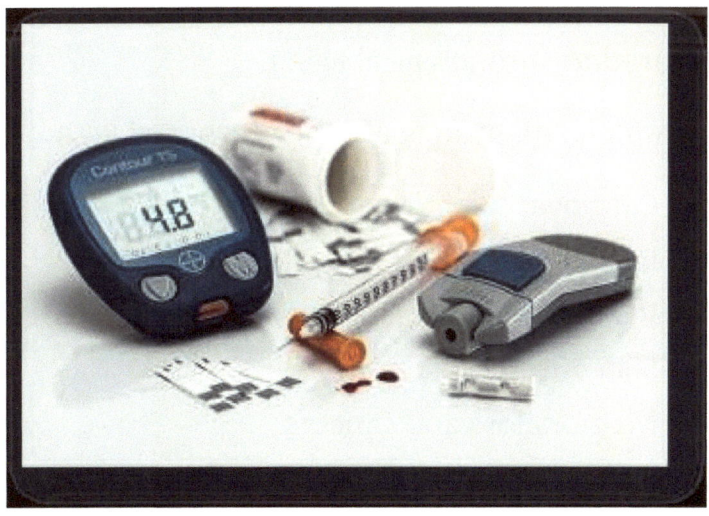

Certainly, many of the complications of diabetes can make us older than our years. Statistics show that diabetic patients live four to eight years less than those people who do not have the disease. So, diabetes makes them older than their years.

Compounding Factors

Complicating this is that diabetes is rarely the only 'age-related' condition a person is diagnosed with. The same environmental and lifestyle factors which brought about an incidence of type 2 diabetes is very likely to have triggered other diseases or conditions.

Over time, a person will often be diagnosed with a cluster of age-related diseases in common with diabetes. Although attributed to aging, all of them contribute to advanced apparent aging as compared to chronological aging.

For example, many may also be diagnosed with:

- Cardiovascular diseases
- Impotence
- Vision and hearing problems
- Skin diseases
- Memory loss and cancers.

Some of these diseases and conditions can be traced to environmental causes such as toxins and poisons, such as those that are known to be carcinogenic.

Type 2 Diabetes, Cause and Cure

However, there is an increasing awareness and understanding that the root cause are lifestyle factors, the main one being diet. Lack of exercise can be a contributing factor, but it is secondary to what has been eaten.

The realization that they have been responsible, through past actions, for their condition, can be a shock for a newly-diagnosed diabetic. However, this same knowledge should give hope to them that changing their lifestyle can also bring about a reduction or even a reversal of the disease.

It should also give inspiration to those diagnosed as pre-diabetic, obese or overweight, and to anyone concerned that their current indulgences may lead to type 2 diabetes in their future.

Lifestyle Changes

It is never too late to take personal action to prevent or mitigate the effects of diabetes, but obviously, the earlier changes are made, the less damage will be caused to the body. This will mean increased longevity and quality of life.

It can be extremely difficult for someone diagnosed with type 2 diabetes to overcome the natural resistance to undertaking an exercise program, or making wholesale changes to their diet. The lifestyle choices that led to developing the condition are excessive consumption of simple carbohydrates, usually in conjunction with insufficient physical exertion.

A consequence of this usually an overweight condition, even obesity, which is often a precursor of pre-diabetes, then ultimately diabetes.

This situation occurs over time and although the patient may not be emotionally happy with their state, it can be hard to push through to make the needed lifestyle changes. Habits can be hard to overcome, especially when the choices are between unaccustomed physical exertion and relaxing, or between eating a favorite treat and a less tasty, healthier food choice.

Lifelong Consequences

Once type 2 diabetes has taken hold, some damage to organs and tissue is almost certain. While the diabetes itself may be reduced or reversed, this damage will remain. This can include vision impairment and loss of extremities or limbs due to gangrene.

In conclusion, diabetes certainly takes years off a person's life and can accelerate the aging process. Therefore, it could easily be stated that if you prevent the onset of diabetes in the first place, you could delay the onset of premature aging caused by it.

Aging and Diabetes

Frequent urination, persistent thirst and lethargy are warning signs of diabetes. However, they are often seen as signs of just growing old too!

Many older individuals may remain undiagnosed diabetics for years (as they see their symptoms as just a part of growing old) until their diabetic symptoms become worse.

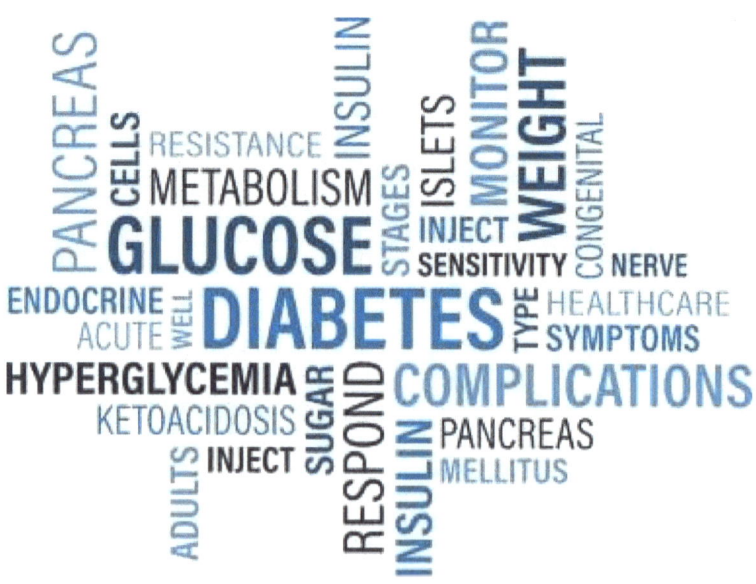

The problem is that irreparable, but avoidable, damage may have already occurred in some parts of the body. Accurate and early diagnosis of type 2 diabetes will be the greatest single factor in reducing the impact of its debilitating symptoms.

Here are some of the health issues that diabetics face, especially as they age.

Problems with Mobility

Physical activity is essential for maintaining optimal health, for diabetics it is especially so. Diabetic individuals who were more athletic when they were younger, could help control their blood glucose levels through regular exercise. However, as they get older, exercising regularly may not be quite as easy.

This means dietary indulgences that in the past might have partly mitigated by exercise, probably now more totally contribute to constantly elevated blood sugar levels. Over time, with reduced activity, this pre-diabetic condition will more likely develop into full-blown type 2 diabetes.

Overcoming Inertia

It can be challenging to change the sedentary behaviors of a lifetime and replace them with a regular and effective exercise routine. Any exercise program will cause discomfort initially. This must be overcome until the routine becomes a new and healthy habit. Learn the difference between discomfort and pain.

Any changes to exercise patterns should be made gradually. Start small and increase the effort as your fitness levels improve. Exertion should cause an increase in heart and breathing rates, but should not cause distress or undue fatigue.

Stop before this happens and set your sights lower to begin with. Ideally, an individualized exercise plan should be made with the help of a health care professional or fitness expert familiar with geriatric health.

Exercises that will prove to be the most beneficial for elderly diabetics include light weight training and walking. These can be undertaken with little equipment and the effort easily scaled to suit current fitness levels.

Aggravated Health Conditions

Many seniors may have bone and joint disorders, which can certainly hamper their ability to exercise.

Another problem for diabetics is that of having a higher risk of heart disease. It is recommended that an exercise stress test be taken before performing any strenuous exercise or physical activity.

Increased Risk of Fractures

Although fractures and the tendency to fall are high among the aged population, being diagnosed with diabetes can raise the risk even higher.

Diabetics may suffer from leg cramps due to excessive urination which causes the person to become dehydrated, but leg cramps can also be a sign of damage to the nerves known as 'diabetic neuropathy'. This is caused from blood sugar levels being persistently too high.

Diabetic symptoms - the shakiness, imbalance, lack of co-ordination and weakness, all increase their likelihood of falling and suffering bone fractures.

Drug Interactions

Diabetics are usually prescribed more than just one type of medicine, especially aging patients. They may need to take several medications to be able to manage their multiple medical conditions.

Thus, their risk of experiencing side effects and adverse drug interactions are also higher. It is vitally important that any unanticipated symptoms are immediately reported to the doctor and/or pharmacist.

Being diabetic, regardless of age, is not easy. Advancing age will of course add another layer of difficulty. However, mindful and determined effort by the patient, under the guidance of health professionals, can greatly reduce the impact of diabetic symptoms and enhance quality of life.

The Importance of Sun Exposure

as We Age

We often talk about eating whole foods and staying active to achieve optimal health, but many of us tend to overlook the importance of sun exposure as we age.

This is not entirely the fault of the individual, as many health campaigns, focused on reducing skin cancer, have created a near-phobia of the sun in many people.

 As with most things related to health, balance is required. It is not wise to have skin exposed to the sun for long periods in the middle part of the day when burning is likely.

It is just as un-wise to avoid the sun altogether, as our bodies rely on the sun's rays for our adequate vitamin D requirements. Getting out in the sun and soaking up vitamin D is very important for keeping our bodies healthy against many age-related diseases.

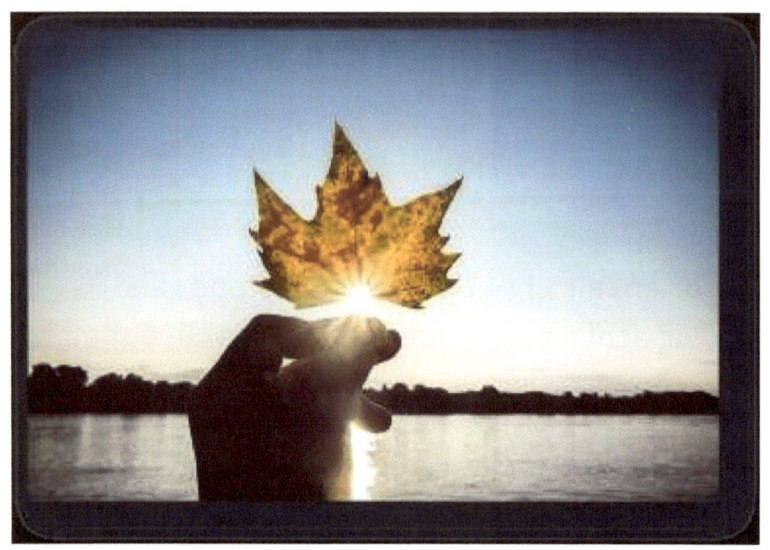

For those concerned about getting skin cancer, experts from 'Cancer Research UK' state that the amount of exposure it takes for an individual to get enough vitamin D is less than the amount that will cause skin cancer.

Many people rely on foods they eat as their source of vitamin D, and that's good too, however, dietary sources can barely provide 400 units of vitamin D, whereas exposure to sunlight can easily give us more than 20,000 units per day.

Lack of Exposure to Sunlight

The importance of vitamin D cannot be overemphasized especially as we age.

Many experts have expressed their concern about the elderly who don't get enough exposure to sunlight every day and are therefore lacking vitamin D. Some stay indoors because their medical condition prevents them from being mobile, others prefer to be outdoors, but are all covered up from head to toe.

Many people today, young and old, do not have enough vitamin D in their system.

This is why many experts urge people to not be totally covered up when exposing their body to the sun. Even having your forearms exposed for 20 minutes, before the heat of the day sets in, is enough for your body to absorb its needed vitamin D.

Sunshine for Brain and Heart Health

The health of the brain and heart will benefit from exposure to sunlight. This is because they both require vitamin D. Medical studies have shown that people who have Alzheimer's disease were found to be 70 to 90% vitamin D deficient.

Experts also found that increasing the levels of vitamin D through sunlight exposure, and from dietary sources, helped improve cognitive functioning among the elderly who were diagnosed with Alzheimer's and of course in those who didn't.

Sunshine for the Prevention of Metabolic Syndrome

Vitamin D deficiency increases the risk of metabolic syndrome. Lacking exposure to sunlight is one of the factors attributed to increasing incidences of so-called 'age-related' diseases.

One study showed that 94% of study participants, aged between 50 to 70 years of age and who were living in China, were vitamin D deficient and 42% of those people were diagnosed with metabolic syndrome.

Similar rates have been subsequently observed among American and British populations.

Osteoporosis

A great concern of aging is that of osteoporosis. Advice in the past has strongly promoted calcium to the exclusion of all else for bone strength.

Modern research shows that in the absence of both vitamin D and the mineral magnesium, calcium intake is wasted, as the body cannot utilize calcium for bone growth without them.

Therefore, don't be afraid of the sun, just be smart about when and for how long when it comes to exposure. Your health depends upon it.

Digestive Health Issues as People Age

One very common health issue among the aging population is digestive health. The body changes as we age and our digestive system is quite often affected in the process. Here are a few problems many face as the years progress.

Slow Bowel Function

A sluggish bowel increases the risk of being constipated. Much of the work inside the colon involves coordinated contraction of the smooth muscles that are in the gut. For this coordinated contraction to function smoothly, an individual must eat a healthy diet, drink plenty of water and partake in physical activity.

The problem is, as people age they tend to let at least one of these 3 things slide. If it is spending less time doing physical activities, the result can be a sluggish digestive system. This 'cause' has an 'effect'. Their stools may then be harder to pass.

This isn't something they have to live with! A sluggish colon can be improved with the help of an increased intake of foods that are rich in soluble fiber, increased fluid intake and regular exercise.

Diverticulosis

Although not just an 'old-age' diseases, many older adults suffer from a susceptibility to diverticulosis. This is when small pouches start to develop in the lining of a person's colon. These diverticula pouches will eventually lead to digestive problems such as constipation.

In addition, when the pouches become inflamed the person may suffer from abdominal pain, tenderness and fever. Some people who have this condition may even suffer from rectal bleeding.

Not Getting Enough Fluid

Regardless of age, we need to drink plenty of water to avoid constipation. However, fluid intake may become a problem for older adults, especially when they start taking medications that have diuretic effects such as those commonly prescribed for heart failure and high blood pressure.

These diuretics help reduce blood pressure by allowing the body to lose excess fluids through frequent urination.

As a consequence, some people reduce their fluid intake in order to avoid making frequent visits to the bathroom, thereby increasing their risk of becoming dehydrated. This is when constipation and other digestive problems can start to occur.

Increased Food Sensitivity

One common complaint associated with aging is the increased sensitivity to some spicy foods, coffee or alcoholic beverages. Some people find they are no longer capable of tolerating the same kinds of foods as they did when they were younger. They often experience a 'gassy' feeling, along with other digestive problems such as dyspepsia and heart burn.

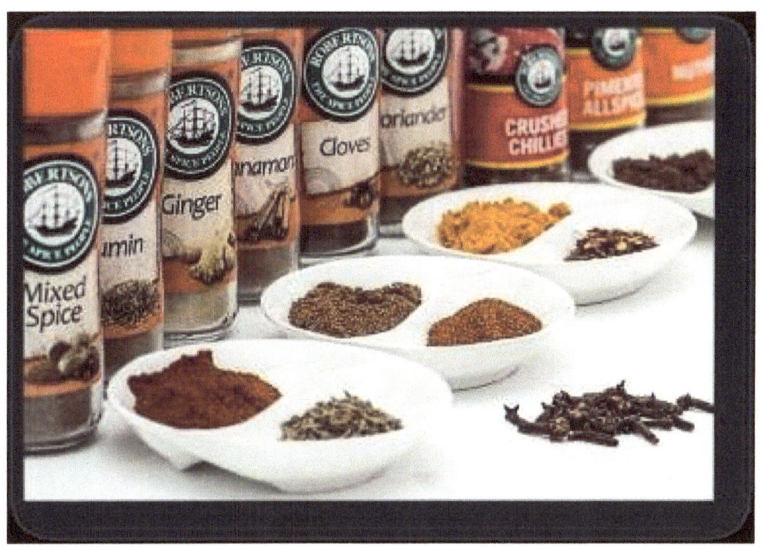

Medications

Medications are another problem for digestive health. As people age, there is a greater tendency to take medications which increases the risk of suffering from their side effects, one of which can be constipation. Narcotic pain relievers, aspirin, NSAIDs and other over-the-counter drugs may cause constipation, GI bleeding and upset stomach.

Thyroid Problems and Diabetes

Diabetes and thyroid problems are a few examples of illnesses that may occur in some people as they age.

Unfortunately, these conditions trigger the occurrence of digestive problems such as diarrhea and constipation. Diabetes is also known to slow down the process of emptying the stomach, resulting in increased digestive discomforts.

Being Overweight

Increased weight also increases the risk of experiencing heart burn and acid reflux. This is because as more weight is gained, more abdominal fat can push the stomach up, resulting in feelings of discomfort.

Screening Tests for Early Cancer Detection

Cancer is an insidious disease and as people age, many are afraid of developing cancer. As a person ages, their risk increases, unless lifestyle modifications and other positive interventions are undertaken to prevent it.

There are many reasons as to why this can happen. One is, as a person gets older, their immune system may have a reduced capability to respond efficiently to pathogens and preventing the formation of a tumor. This occurrence is what experts refer to as immune-senescence, and one of its consequences is the higher risk for developing diseases such as cancer.

Cancer starts to occur when cells in any parts of the body become abnormal. These abnormal cells eventually form into a mass of tissue which is referred to as malignant or cancerous tumor.

Apart from optimizing your health through a healthy diet, exercise and avoidance of toxins, experts say the greatest factor in cancer survival is early detection.

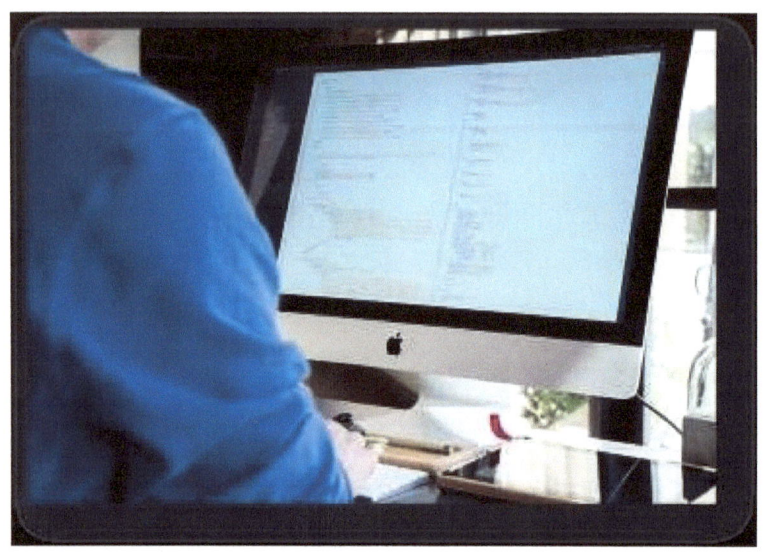

Cancer Screening Tests

The following is a list of screening tests that can be scheduled on a regular basis to help prevent or detect cancer in its earliest stage.

Breast Cancer

- Mammogram - This is an x-ray of the breast. It is designed to detect any cancerous tumors that may be too small to feel by hand.
- Clinical Breast Exam - A health care professional checks the breasts and

underarms for the existence of lumps and other unusual changes.

Colorectal Cancer

- Fecal Occult Blood Test - This test requires the patient to submit a stool sample which is sent to the lab for examination. The presence of hidden blood in the person's stool can be a sign of cancer. Doctors recommend undergoing a fecal occult blood test at least once a year or every two years if the person is 50 years of age or above. Research shows that colorectal cancer is mostly diagnosed among individuals who are 50 years old and above.

- Sigmoidoscopy - A thin, flexible tube will be used by the doctor to look inside the person's lower part of the colon and rectum to check for any presence of abnormal growths. If this test is done every five years the risk of getting colorectal cancer can be reduced.

- Colonoscopy - Doctors recommend that people undergo a colonoscopy once every ten years.

This test works a lot like the sigmoidoscopy, the only difference is that a colonoscopy allows the doctor to see the entire colon of the person.

Prostate Cancer

- Digital Rectal Exam - This exam allows the doctor to insert his gloved finger into the person's rectum to be able to feel the prostate. If the doctor detects some hard or lumpy areas he will then conduct further examinations to be able to confirm if the patient has cancer.
- PSA or Prostate Specific Antigen Test - This is when the amount of PSA is measured using blood samples. If the person's PSA is found to be higher than normal, then it is also possible that prostate cancer cells are present. Having high levels of PSA is one indicator that the person has a problem in his prostate.

If you are diagnosed with cancer, it is always wise to get a second opinion. That way you may also be given different treatment options.

Growing older does not mean getting cancer, however taking precautionary steps, such as making healthy lifestyle choices and taking regular screening tests, is a great start to reducing your risk and for the doctors to make an early diagnosis.

Conclusion

Growing old is not a disease, or even a condition –
it is a consequence of the inevitable aging process.
While some events and circumstances are
unavoidable, many issues relating to our health is
very much "reap what you sow".

Whatever stage of life you are at now, it only goes
in one direction. Make positive changes now so
that in the future you don't look back and say "if
only".

Other Relevant Books By This Author

https://www.createspace.com/ 6988329

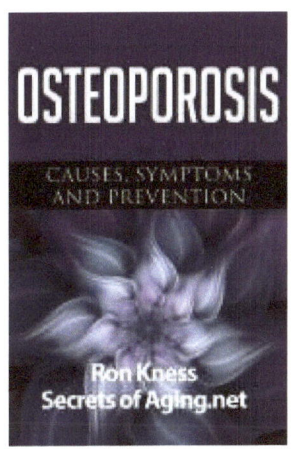

Osteoporosis: Causes, Symptoms and Prevention

We all want to be less vulnerable to bone breakage as we age. We also want to reduce the risk of falling, breaking a hip and ultimately risk losing our independence because the fracture doesn't heal correctly. And we want to prevent and preserve bone density for as long as possible!

We can achieve ALL of these goals with the newest release from Ron Kness called *Osteoporosis - Causes, Symptoms And Prevention*. Based on these exciting teachings, you will learn about all the dramatic benefits of good bone health, performing weight-bearing exercising and eating healthy foods as a way to preserve bone density.

This book is built around a very clear, concept: maintain bone density and bone health as part of a healthy lifestyle for as long as possible.

It's not just about keeping bones healthy as we age. Having great bone health is linked to being active, exercising and eating foods that support bone health. This is because eating the right foods and doing "weight-bearing" activities promotes bone density replenishment and reduces bone density loss.

In this book, we look at all the ways you can improve your own bone health, starting with not losing bone density in the first place.

This book will also look at the many other steps that can be taken to support this goal, from making healthy lifestyle choices that support bone health as early as possible, to not smoking or abuse drinking, eating healthy foods and exercising. The choices you make about healthy food, strength training and beneficial supplements that support good bone health have an impact on your bone health.

In *Osteoporosis - Causes, Symptoms And Prevention*, we'll cover all the bases, giving you everything you need to know to preserve, and in some cases restore, bone density.

https://www.createspace.com/6155567

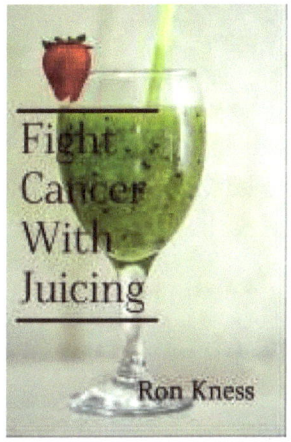

Fight Cancer With Juicing: Use the
Power of Natural Juice to Help
Prevent and Fight Off Cancer

Juicing is a healthy practice that has allowed millions of people to boost their nutrition. Juicing fruits and vegetables provides you important antioxidants, which scavenge for oxygen free radicals that can damage cellular structures, including DNA. When DNA is damaged, it can result in mutations that lead to cancer.

Well-balanced nutrition from a variety of healthy whole foods helps support and maintain on-going good health, and experts agree that nutrition plays a key role in preventing chronic and terminal illness.

When juicing is done right, that is when the majority of your juice blends is comprised of vegetables and very low sugar fruit, you can easily boost your nutritional intake thereby improving your health and lower your risks for cancer.

This book gives you the information needed to not only help prevent cancer in the first place, but to help fight it naturally if you already have it.

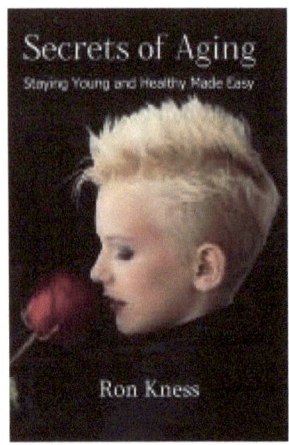

[Secrets of Aging: Staying Young and Healthy Made Easy](#)

We all want to be young and beautiful regardless of age. We also want to be healthy. And we want to minimize the effects of aging!

We can achieve ALL of these goals with my newest release *Secrets of Aging*. Based on these exciting teachings, you will learn about all the dramatic benefits of staying young looking by using a good skincare and beauty regimen and living a healthy lifestyle as a way of staying younger looking than your real age.

This book is built around a very clear, concept: look young and be healthy for as long as possible.

It's not just about methods used to reduce, and in some cases reverse, the effects of aging. Having great looks and health as we age is linked to living a healthy lifestyle and taking of ourselves.

This is possible with the use of proven anti-aging methods and products.

In this book, we look at all of the ways you can improve your own looks and health as you age, starting with a healthy lifestyle.

This book will also look at the many other steps that can be taken to support this goal, from eating healthy foods and using a skincare maintenance program, to dressing, using make-up and wearing a hairstyle appropriate for people your age.

The choices you make now about taking care of your body both inside and out has an impact on your looks and health as you age!

In *Secrets of Aging*, we'll cover all the bases, giving you everything you need to know about using anti-aging tips and techniques to stay young and healthy for as long as possible.

About the Author

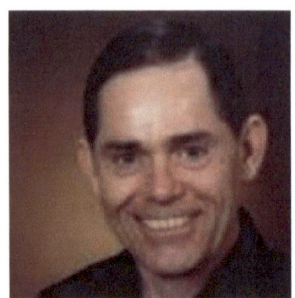

I grew up in Central Minnesota, where my parents owned and operated a fishing resort. Once out of high school I tried a couple of semesters of college, only to quit halfway through the Spring term; I decided at that time that college wasn't for me.

I eventually went back to college 15 years later on the GI Bill and by taking classes at night and on weekends earned my Bachelor's degree in Business Administration.

My interest in writing started because of a teacher that taught me a new way to look at writing. Fast forward about 40 years and I now have published over 125 books on Amazon for Kindle, CreateSpace and other publishing platforms.

While most of my books are on health and fitness in general, as I age (now 65) at the time of this writing) my topics of interest are geared toward aging baby boomers and older.

Besides my own writing, I also ghostwrite ebooks, books, reports, articles, blogs and do Kindle conversions for clients on a variety of topics.

Today my wife and I are retired from our careers and live in Gold Canyon, AZ. I now write as a retirement business where you'll find me happily sitting in my office typing away on my laptop as I work on my next book or ghostwriting project . . . that is if we are not traveling on a cruise ship - our new-found mode of travel.

www.ingramcontent.com/pod-product-compliance
Lightning Source LLC
Chambersburg PA
CBHW040311010626
45792CB00022B/132